Prologue

This is a story about Luna and her struggles with life after a medically induced opioid addiction. It explains how not all addictions come from bad choices, although most do, some come from necessity and the need to be **pain-free.** Follow me on her journey as you get a first hand glimpse into her pain and pleasure receptors and learn how easily you can be pulled into the grip of addiction. Luna never had an easy life but all of her struggles shaped her into the wonderful and loving woman she is today. She stands as a strong and proud human, not to be frowned upon by society and shamed as a recovering addict.

How do I know this, you may ask?
I know because I AM LUNA - and this is my story.

TRIGGER WARNING:

This book contains first-hand depictions of child abuse and rape.

Introduction

It was a bitter & cold December morning. A Saturday, if that matters. Winters have been more and more unpredictable as the years pass by. This time last year she was sipping her coffee on the back porch, wrapped in a light throw, watching the neighbor kids play in the front yard across the road. This wasn't an "outside" type of morning though and Luna was bundled up in her cozy blanket on the sofa, piping hot mug of coffee in hand, waiting for inspiration to swirl through her somewhat morbid mind. You see, Luna wasn't really an outdoorsy type of girl anymore. She spent most of her "non-working" time in her home reading, writing and watching whatever piqued her interest on the television. She still worked but could only take office jobs now. Chronic pain and anxiety had taken control of her life and held her in its vise-like talons for quite a while now, well, ever since "it" happened. As she sips her morning brew, *Luna recounts the sequence of events that led her to live the life she now lives.*

The day started as any other day, it was Tuesday, she remembers because it was St. Patrick's day and she was rushing around that morning to find something in her wardrobe that was green. David was grabbing bookbags and ushering the kids in the car to take them to school as Luna started getting ready for work. She kissed the kids and David, wished them all a good day and ran back upstairs to finish up. Fifteen minutes later, Luna grabs her purse and a banana, then locks the door behind her. She gets into her shiny new Monte Carlo SS and makes the thirty minute drive to work. She had recently taken a job managing a home healthcare company and had over sixty employees that she had to keep track of, literally. She did all the scheduling for the CNA's and the nurses and made sure all of the patients were seen on the days and times that were allotted. She also did all the hiring, HR, and state required documentation that the company needed to keep on file in order to stay in business.

It was a very mentally taxing job to say the least and at the end of the day, Luna was beyond exhausted and started her car for the thirty minute trek home.

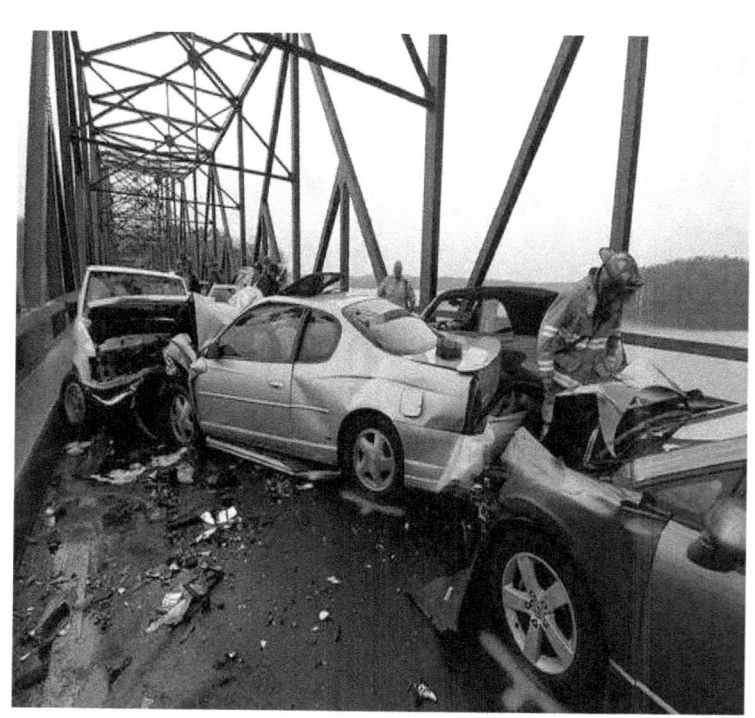
8

Chapter 1   (The Accident)

Luna slams both feet down on the brake pedal and swerves out into the other lane to avoid the collision and crashes head-on into a truck. It felt like she had just hit a brick wall and time immediately stood still. She sits there stunned. She's gasping for breath in the aftermath of the tangled steel of wreckage, dazed and confused with smoke filling the cab of the car. The tangy stench of sodium azide lodged in her nostrils from the airbags deployment, Luna knew somehow that her life would never be the same. With ringing ears and blurry vision, she tried to assess the situation but everything was so foggy and her brain was not sending the signals to her arms to move. Shock had set in. Suddenly there is a man yelling something at her from her window but she can't understand what he's saying and is desperately trying to get the door open because she can see flames and billowing smoke coming from what's left of her engine.

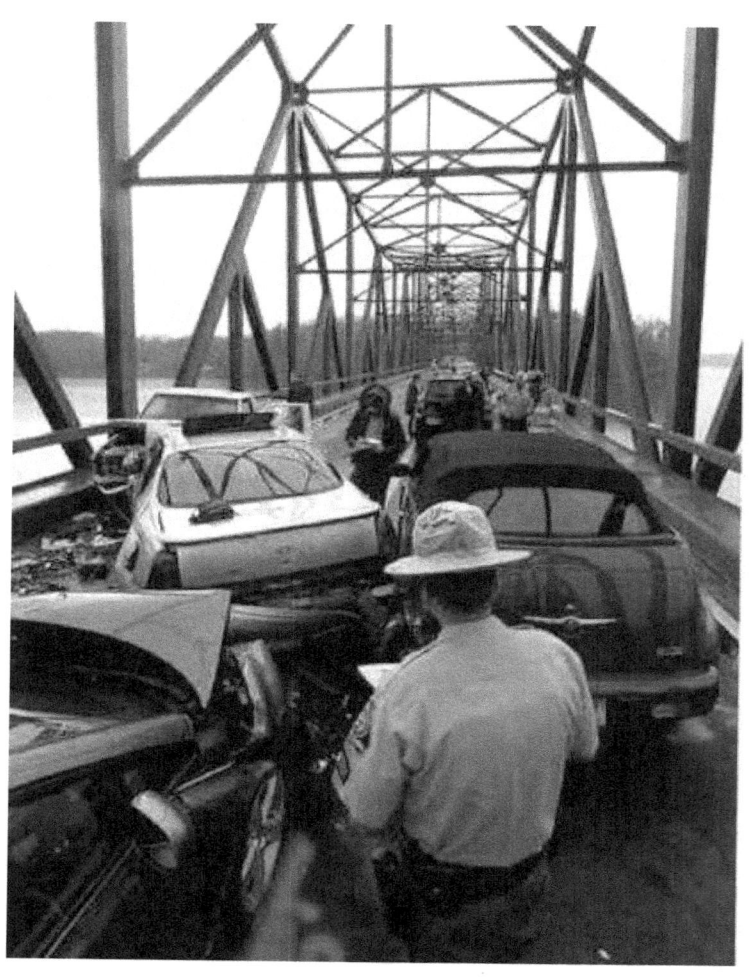

She jumps as the driver side door is ripped open and strong arms reach inside, grabbing her and pulling her from the fiery crash, carrying Luna to the other side of the bridge. Still very shaken and confused, she looks up into the eyes of this stranger and sees that it's the same mocha brown eyes she stared straight into in the split second before her Monte Carlo slammed into his Chevy S10. Crying now, she frantically asks over and over again if he is ok even though she can see the same blank and pained expression on his face that she must have on hers. They sit together on the cross-ties of the bridge as the paramedics and fire trucks are arriving "shit!" she exclaims, she forgot that her car was on fire! She tries to get up and run to the car to grab her belongings and that's when the pain hits. Searing pain rushes to all extremities and knocks her back a step as the paramedics grab her to keep her from falling. Crying uncontrollably now, she could barely talk to tell them what hurt and all she kept saying was "*im broken, im broken*" and then the shortness of breath took over and it was all she could do to even breathe, much less talk.

They carefully place her neck in a brace as they are lifting her to the gurney and into the ambulance, she is gripping something tight in her right hand and feels the EMT trying to take it as she grips it tighter and tighter before realizing it's her phone. Relaxing her grip, she asks the young man to please call her boyfriend and let him know where they are taking her. She was on her way home and he will worry if she's not there soon. A wide-eyed nod meets her stare as he takes the phone and makes the call. She is so sleepy and they keep screaming in her face to stay awake but the darkness is calming, comforting and it beckons her with sweet release.

STAY AWAKE MA'AM! CAN YOU TELL ME YOUR NAME? Drifting in and out of consciousness, Luna thinks *"Jeeze, why is he screaming at me like that and why can I not breathe?"* Everything is an echo. "Ouch!" She is pulled back from the darkness by needles probing, prodding her arms, an EMT on each floppy arm. "We have to place two IV's ma'am, in case you need surgery when we get there." Nodding, Luna asks "what's wrong with my legs?" With the IV's placed, the young man starts from her ankles, cutting her pants off in silent concentration and all Luna could think is "*oh God, i'm not wearing any underwear today.*" She looks up and tells him to please not cut all the way up and he replies that he was so very sorry but he had to. She knows she should not even worry, but *she does*. He grabs something from behind her head and places a sheet over her middle section as he continues to cut through her favorite work pants. When finished, he starts in on her top and begins cutting the fabric, *even though it's a button-up blouse.* He places the stickers for the EKG leads across her chest and on her upper stomach which has already started to turn a different shade from the bruising. He then calls on his radio to the hospital to confirm their arrival and to have a trauma team ready and waiting. Again, Luna asks "please, can you tell me what's wrong with my legs?" He looks at her and said "ma'am, i'm really not supposed to say but it appears that either one or both of your feet and possibly ankles also are broken, but I can't tell any more than that without x-rays and they will do those as soon as we arrive at the hospital" Nodding again, she says in a whisper "my name is Luna" then she closed her eyes and tried to focus on breathing. Something is wrong though, she can't seem to get a full breath into her lungs and tells the young EMT this. He pulls out his stethoscope and listens for a minute, a look of concern on his face, he grabs the oxygen from somewhere overhead and places it over Luna's mouth and nose, she knows somewhere in the back of her mind that she is in shock and Luna was now genuinely terrified.

They arrive at the hospital, sirens blaring in typical emergent-style fashion and all of a sudden there are doctors and nurses all around her. Faces blurry and hurried, she is whisked to the trauma center and evaluated from head to toe. Tubes and wires are placed all over her body and she feels like an alien laying there while they are poking and prodding her already bruised and broken bones.

Doctors giving orders to nurses, hospital staff flurrying around the room with supplies. Luna watches, eyes darting back and forth in fear. She wondered why everyone was talking to each other but no one was talking to her. *Was she that bad off? Is this really happening?* It felt like a dream and she was on the outside looking in, watching a badly scripted horror show. She is left alone for a few minutes while the nurse leaves to search for supplies to place a catheter, Luna hears a familiar voice and looks beyond the half pulled curtain to see the man she hit. He is sitting on the edge of a hospital bed and a doctor is tending to his foot. He looks up and they make eye contact and he mouths "are you ok?" Luna nods and frowns before mouthing back "I'm so sorry" and she really truly was.

Her mind was going non-stop as scenario after scenario played out in her head of what she could've done differently. It all happened **so** fast though. She watches as the doctor talks to the man and then turns and points in her direction. The man nodded, the doctor jotted down a note on his pad and walked away.

Luna, not wanting to invade his privacy any more than she feels she already has, lays back in her bed and closes her eyes again as she prays that he does not sue her.

The nurse comes back and places the catheter and lets her know that a trauma team member is on the way up to take her down for a CT scan and x-rays but before leaving the room she looks at Luna and say's "you're lucky, you know" confused, Luna asks "why?" and the nurse replies "I don't know how you did it but you don't have a single scratch or mark on your face" and she smiled again before saying "you're going to be ok hun" and walked away. Luna's hands, covered in tubes and wires, go to her face for the first time as she explores the contours in awe. She remembers the moment just before impact when her hands, having a will of their own, left the steering wheel and pressed themselves to her face. She ponders the reason and it wasn't vanity, she just did not want to see what was about to happen. Shaking her head, Luna closes her eyes and replays the scene over and over, not because she wanted to, it just would not go away. Everything was black and white, projector-style and slowed down like she was in an old film noir. Startled back to reality again, the trauma team arrives and she is taken down for x-rays and CT scan. The pain returns with a vengeance as she thinks "*why do they have to twist and turn my body like that, can't the machine see everything, don't they know how bad this hurts?*" Tears spill down her cheeks as the pain quickens to the point of screaming, but she does not scream. It feels virtually impossible when she still can't even breathe a full breath into her hollow lungs. The tech takes her back up to her room to wait on the doctor and just a short amount of time passes before the doctor sends a nurse in to give her some pain relief. *Finally,* the pain ebbs down to a low hum and is tolerable enough for Luna to close her eyes and try to sleep. Sleep is a fickle bedfellow though as the doctors and nurses are in and out of the room, talking, barking orders and turning her this way and the other. Just as the darkness begins to take hold, a doctor comes in and tells her that her left lung has collapsed which is why she is having trouble breathing, the medical term is pneumothorax, and they need another scan to see if it will reinflate on its own or if they will need to insert a chest tube. Luna is whisked away to be scanned and then back up to the room again. Upon returning to her room she is met by her boyfriend David, who was, to say the least, frantic. After telling him what she could remember about the accident, she was finally able to fall asleep for a while. While she was sleeping, the doctor came in and talked to David.

He informed him that "Luna had a tear in her lung, most likely from the seatbelt pressure during impact, causing it to collapse, however, the tear was small and would not require a chest tube and will heal with oxygen therapy, rest and time.
In addition to both deep and superficial bumps and bruises that will eventually heal, she has also broken and displaced just about every bone in her right foot. Initially, we thought that she had broken both feet but we are not seeing any

fractures on the left side, just a fair amount of swelling from the tissue damage. You may notice that her knees are the size of grapefruits but we cannot see any breaks there, only swelling and more tissue damage. Her whole body will eventually be black and blue, just a heads up. We want to refer her to an orthopedic specialist for her foot but we do need to keep her in CCU for the next few days at the least to monitor the damage to her lung and we can also help with pain control while she is here. We will contact the surgeon and he can stop in to see her on his rounds." David thanks the doctor and returns to his chair, waiting for Luna to awaken.

Chapter 2 (Pain & Paradise)

Upon awakening, Luna noticed that she was in a different room than the one she fell asleep in. David was there, and so were her children Zoe and Blake. The looks of concern and fear on their faces immediately triggered the waterworks and she motioned them over for hugs and reassurance. She could tell that they were scared but they were "mama's brave little soldiers" and were trying their best to hide it. She smiled and told them everything would be ok as she looked at David, silently questioning her response. He raised his brow and shrugged, hugging the kids and ushering them out to the vending machine in the waiting area.

David returned a few minutes later without the kids in tow and sat down to tell her what the doctor had told him while she slept. Luna was relieved that the damage to her lung was minimal and would heal without surgery but very concerned about her foot. With IV pain medications flowing through her system she could barely tell that she was even hurt.

A million questions started tumbling in her head as she asked David if he had called her boss, work, omg would she get fired? She had only had her job for about four months and knew this was going to inconvenience her boss and the company she was managing. How long would she be out? When will the surgeon see her? Was this considered a major surgery? She has no health insurance, will they even do the surgery if she's uninsured? Has anyone heard anything about the young man she had collided with? Was he ok? Ugh, this was just too much for her battered body and mind to process right now she thought as she felt herself drifting back to sleep.

The beeping and buzzing machines hooked to her body roused her from sleep some time later. She looked at the clock on the wall, it read 1:37. She wondered if it was day or night as there were no windows in the CCU rooms. She pressed her call button and a nurse came in with her caddy of supplies and let her know it was night and she would be her nurse until the next shift arrived at 7am.

She told her that her name was Holly and Luna could call on her if she needed anything. She took down her vitals and pressed another syringe full of *"sweet, sweet bliss"* into her IV, asked if her pain level was tolerable and walked back out of the room leaving Luna alone to rest. But rest would not come. Too many thoughts invaded her mind. She was afraid. She laid there for what felt like an eternity listening to the steady hum and beeping of the monitors as her mind wandered back to all of the unanswered questions she had earlier. *What was she going to do? Her boss was going to have a coronary. What will happen if she loses her job?* Shaking her head as if to shake away the unwelcome thoughts, she settled the best she could into the hospital bed and let the pain medications take her back to the darkness that she *preferred*.

In the morning, Luna awakens to David and some close friends of theirs who wanted to come check on her. She was really thankful for their concern but at the same time, wished David had given her a heads up because after everything she'd been through over the last twenty four hours, she knew she must look like she had wrestled with a bobcat. Still, Luna smiled and thanked them for coming and answered all the questions they had concerning the wreck. They did not stay long thankfully and soon after they left two officers knocked lightly, walked in and introduced themselves. They were investigating the crash and needed information from her regarding her side of the story, auto insurance information and took a picture of her drivers license to have on file for the report. She was able to ask the officer if he knew how the other driver was and if he was ok. They said that they had just come from his room and he was doing fine, that he had suffered a broken foot and a concussion. She was most relieved that his injuries were no more severe than hers and at least got one of her pressing questions answered.

The officers informed her that there were more than just the two of them involved in the accident. It was actually documented as a five car pile up. Shocked, she asked what exactly happened and from the investigation they were able to tell her that it originated from a single stalled car on the bridge. The car in front of Luna actually hit the stalled car and Luna swerved to avoid the accident and hit the truck head on. The car behind Luna saw her swerve and followed suit only to crash into the rear of her car. Trying to relive the scenario out in her mind, she shuddered. She had no idea she had even been hit in the rear. After asking if the other parties were ok and reassured that they were, the officers finished their questions, left her a card with a case number to call later to get a copy of the police report for her insurance company and left. Letting out a huge breath of air that she didn't even realize she had been holding, Luna looked at David and said rather sheepishly "I'm in trouble huh?" David smiled and replied "go big or go home right?" She wished she could laugh at that little retort but her pain medication must be wearing off and her foot was starting to throb so badly that all she could do was burst into tears.

David came to the bed and held her while she broke down and picked up the call button and called the nurse for another dose of meds. When the nurse arrived she saw that she was crying and went ahead and gave her another full dose of dilaudid, asked David to take a break and let Luna get some rest while the medication took effect. He kissed her and told her he would be back later with the kids and Luna, being both physically and emotionally drained, once again *drifted off into the darkness and oh, how she loved it there.*

She was awakened some time later, *as if time had any meaning anymore*, to a nurse shaking her and telling her to "wake up and put this oxygen mask on" Startled, she asked what was happening and the nurse told her that she was not breathing well and needed to wear the oxygen to get her level back up as it had dropped down into the fifties. Luna, having some medical training, knew that this was not good so she struggled to wake up better and focus on breathing in as much oxygen as she could to get that back to a good level. The nurse stood there over her for quite some time monitoring her oxygen intake and vitals while Luna breathed in and breathed out rhythmically and when the level reached ninety seven the nurse turned down the output and placed a nasal cannula in her nose and told her she wanted her to wear it for the night as the dilaudid that they gave her earlier was suppressing her respiratory system. When the nurse left, Luna glanced at the clock and saw that it was close to five o'clock and wondered where David and the kids were.

She didn't have to wonder very long as a few minutes later they all walked into the room with bright smiles, cards that the kids had made and balloons with well wishes written all over the shiny aluminum type material. Smiles were replaced with looks of concern as they all saw the oxygen tube in her nose.

Luna assured them all was ok and they're just making her wear it because of the effects of the medication and immediately, she saw the smiles return to their precious faces, which really, was all that mattered to her at that moment. Plenty of hugs and giggles came that evening and her heart was happy even though her body was betraying her. They had brought themselves and her some dinner so that she didn't have to eat the bland hospital food and they sat there and enjoyed a meal together in her little room that seemed to be home for now and it was the most "normal" Luna had felt in two days. *Two days*, she thought to herself, *why did it feel like she had been here for a week?* With a wistful sigh and a full stomach she settled into her hospital bed with her children on each side and David in the chair by the bed. She relaxed and let the drugs work their magic as she drifted into the darkness again.

When she woke up next, it was morning. She could tell by the changing of the shift nurses and rang for one to come help her try to get out of bed and into the chair that David had occupied last night. They must have left last night after she passed out on them. She hoped he was doing well alone with the kids as she was normally the one who tended to their needs. David was not their father and even though she trusted him, she didn't trust that he was up to date with the in's and outs of their daily routines and lives. *But what could she do?* Deciding not to worry too much about that right now she waited on the nurse to come in and she was able to get up after several failed attempts, and sit in the chair. Breakfast came with a "thunk" of the tray on the bedside table as the dietary aide hurried off without a word. Lifting the lid, she could only wrinkle her nose and pray that it tasted better than it smelled. It wasn't long after breakfast that the searing pain decided to make itself known and Luna called the nurse again and asked for more medication.

Today's nurse, Kimberly, eyed the clock and told her that she still had another hour before she could give her the strong stuff but offered something for breakthrough pain which Luna was thankful for and accepted but was really looking forward to the dose of the stronger stuff so her pain would go away completely. Looking down at her right leg with her fat knees and swollen, blackened foot, she wondered when the surgeon would make it by and let her know when she could have her surgery, and if it were possible with no insurance. She thought to herself, *my god, what will happen if I can't have the surgery? The doctor said that every bone in there was broken.* Luna sighed and grabbed the remote to the tiny television that was mounted on the wall and tried to distract her mind from the pain and the fears that haunted her waking thoughts. Kimberly finally walked in with the *blessed syringe* she had been longing for and helped get her back to bed before squeezing the "good stuff" into the IV in Luna's arm.

Feeling the familiar warmth spread throughout her body and the comforting weight it bore down on her chest like a weighted blanket, Luna was greeted by darkness once again as she closed her eyes and said hello to her new best friend. Dilaudid.

Her dreams were always lucid when the medication seared through her bloodstream, Everything was full of color and adventure. Not at all comparable to the drab off-white walls of the hospital room where all you can hear are the beeps and boops of the medical equipment and the nurses barking orders to the CNA's down the halls. No, here in her dilaudid utopia, the birds were singing and the sky was azure blue with no clouds in sight. She could practically taste the colors. The sun was shining, reflecting off of the water of what could only be Lake Serenity. *This was her paradise.*

Chapter 3 (Fear & Addiction)

Hello Luna, Im Doctor Sanderson, I'm the orthopedic surgeon that your ER doctor referred you to and I will be evaluating your injury today. Luna's eyes fluttered open and she could now see the face attached to the distant voice that had incorporated itself into her dream world. Blinking a few times to clear the fog, she said hello and asked if he had seen her x-rays and what was his opinion on what, if anything, he had seen thus far. He smiled and told her that he had seen the x-rays and the CT scan and that it appeared that the combination of her foot locked down on the brake pedal and the impact from the crash caused all five of her metatarsal bones to not only break but they had also been displaced. He went on to say that her tarsal bone had a "burst-type" break which looked like someone took a hammer to a rock and smacked it one good time causing it to shatter into so many tiny fragments that it would be quite a task to try and put back together, but he was up for the challenge. He said that the game plan was to wait for the swelling to go down for a couple of days before going in and setting the metatarsals back into place and then, after putting the jigsaw puzzle pieces of her tarsal bone back together he would place a metal plate on top of it and set it all in place with some screws. Piece of cake. The surgery should last about three or four hours and will be done here at the hospital. You should be able to go home the following day. You will be in a hard cast from knee down and non weight-bearing for up to twelve weeks while the bones heal and will be sent home with either a wheelchair, crutches or both. After the twelfth week, providing you are healing well, you will be placed in a walking boot and allowed to bear weight. PT will start then and you will need to work on building your strength back up in that leg. You will one hundred percent lose muscle mass in the leg from lack of use so PT is very important, it's not an option, it's a requirement. Blinking slowly, she asks "will I be able to walk normally after this?" Clasping his hands in front of him, he said "providing the surgery goes as planned and you heal as you should, yes, you should be able to walk normally." He then asked if she had any further questions and she asked when he thought he would be able to operate. He said he was going to book an operating room in two days and they will let her know when it's time. She then told him that she was uninsured and asked if that would be an issue. He turned slowly and replied that yes, that seems to be a slight roadblock. He stated that she could fill out assistance paperwork with the hospital for the use of the operating room and such but that he would have to get back to her with an estimate for the cost of the surgery itself. She thanked him as he was walking away and slumped back into the bed with an exasperated sigh. The wheels in her brain were spinning at a rate that was making her dizzy.

How could she get this paid for? Surely it was not going to be cheap. She was more than likely looking at something in the range of five to ten thousand dollars or so and she knew that they didn't have that kind of money saved. Fighting back tears, she grabs her phone and starts looking for loan companies that may loan that amount or more. Lunch was served with another wordless "thunk' on the bedside table, eyeing it, her stomach turned and she pushed it aside. She had completely lost her appetite and didn't know if it was stress or the medication. She just knew it smelled like roadkill. As she is researching the many different loan companies and the astronomical interest rates they offer, it hits her. Emergency medical aide from Medicaid. She had heard that a friend of hers had used that in the past so she found the number and made the call.

Eureka! Luna was relieved to find out that since she was now technically "unemployed for medical reasons" that she qualified for the emergency medical aide. Relief poured over her like a cold glass of water on a scorching summer day. *Breathe Luna, it's all going to be ok.* It took a while to go through all of the gazillion questions and qualify but she finally got through and thanked the lady on the other end of the call for all of the help she had provided. She then called David and told him the good news.

They would email her the approval letter by the end of the day and the surgery could go on as planned. She could hear the kids in the background and asked how everything was going at home. He said it was all fine, the kids missed me and he would come by again at dinnertime and bring her some decent food. She smiled. More relaxed now, she said her goodbyes and placed the phone on the table by the roadkill, wishing they would come back and take it from the room quickly. Time ticked by slowly as nurses came and went from her room in a steady flow. Pain reared its ugly head again before dinner and the nurse came to the rescue with her *magic syringe* as Luna watched it swoosh out and into the IV, straight into her bloodstream. The now familiar weight pressed down on her chest as her body warmed from the inside out. Blissfully driving out the pain demon that had set up his nest inside her now numbed foot.

Thanking the nurse as she walked away, Luna sat there in wonder as all pain finally subsided and her tired body succumbed to slumber again.

She dreamed in color in her medicine induced utopia. Ferris wheels and cotton candy, people she had never seen and people she had known her whole life we're all there. Everyone was happy and smiling. There was no pain or sadness. *All was good and right in this world.*

"Luna, Luna wake up and look at me for a minute." She pulled herself from her dreamland and opened her eyes. Kimberly was back. *Why was she here? She only works the day shift..* Confused, she tried to crawl through the cobwebs in her head, her mouth felt like she had been sucking on a cotton ball. Reaching for the water on her bedside table and taking a huge gulp, she asks Kimberly what she was doing working so late in the evening. Laughing, Kimberly tells her that it was morning and the night nurse informed her that Luna had slept since early evening. She unwraps and rewraps the blood pressure cuff on her arm as she tells her she even slept through David and the kids visit. She squints, searching through the edges of her mind and tries to remember yesterday evening but she only draws a complete blank. She thinks to herself, *oh man, that stuff is strong*. But she says nothing to Kimberly out of sheer fear that they may agree and lower the dosage and that just can not happen as it seems to be the only thing that takes the unrelenting pain away. As Kimberly finishes up with her morning routine of vitals and urine measurements; breakfast is delivered. Before the dietary aide can plop it on the table, Luna touches her on the arm and asks what day it is. "Its Sunday hun" was her reply as she dropped the tray on the table and hurried away. *Sunday?* she thinks, *the wreck was Tuesday, has it been only 5 days?* Luna eats her breakfast with little to no enthusiasm. Her appetite was almost non-existent and she wondered if she had lost any weight during her stay. Tomorrow is the day she is supposed to have surgery and her anxiety is in the beginning stages of an upward spiral. With her mind still a little groggy, she closes her eyes again and tries to sleep to pass the time. Around lunchtime, David and the kids arrive and she is awakened by their voices invading her dreams. She slowly opens her eyes as they are heavily laden with the throes of sleep and tries to smile but her face does not even feel like the smile exists. *Numb, everything is numb.*

They must have come while she was dreaming and gave her scheduled *"elixyr of the gods"* because she was not feeling an ounce of pain at the moment and it was **glorious**. She turns to David and asks for a wet washcloth to wash the sleepiness from her eyes and notices that they have brought her lunch. Still not hungry but not wanting to appear ungrateful, she takes a few bites and talks with them about their day, asks if they are doing their chores and feeding the cat. She is assured that all is well on the homefront and that eases her mind for now. He brought a newspaper with him and tossed it onto the bed for her to see. Luna's jaw drops to the floor as she sees that the wreck made the front page of the local newspaper. She reads the article and realizes that the EPA had to be called in to try and clear the auto fluids, oil, transmission fluid

etc.. from the lake under the bridge and that made her feel even worse for a moment.
This was apparently a much bigger deal than she had originally thought.

David and the munchkins stay and keep her company with stories from work and school, Luna asks if he had heard from her boss and he had. Thankfully, she still had a job to go back to when all this was finally over and that was the best news she had heard in days. Dinner arrives and David and the kids gather up their belongings and take their leave for the evening and Luna, a little more relaxed with the good news about her job, lays back and lets the medication which is still flowing inside, take her back to the utopia in which she has begun to call *home*.

Chapter 4 (Surgery & Aftermath)

The following morning, Luna is awakened bright and early by Dr. Sanderson. He tells her that surgery is scheduled at noon today and she will be taken down and prepped in about three hours. Looking at his watch, he asks if she had any questions and let her know that someone would be coming by her room in a few minutes with some forms to sign before he hurried away. She picked up her phone and called David to let him know that they now finally have a time and he needed to come soon. With her anxiety now at an all time high, her pain increases ten-fold and she calls for the nurse and asks when her next dose is scheduled. She is told she still has another hour and again, is offered a less effective medication to hold her over. She graciously accepts and they come in and administer it. She barely notices any relief and between the pain and anxiety, Luna can only cry as she waits for administration to come with her surgery paperwork. When they do finally come, she signs all the appropriate forms and begins to get more anxious by the minute as David is still not there. She grabs her phone to call and just as she raises the phone to her ear, he finally walks in.

He walks over to the bed and holds Luna in his arms as she finally loses her shit. The reality of actually having surgery and being put to sleep, her foot sliced open, hit her like a ton of bricks. She was again terrified. The surgery technicians arrive to take Luna to surgery and as they are wheeling her down the hall all she can think is *"what if something goes wrong and I die during surgery?" "Will David care for the kids?"* Once she arrived in the operating room she didn't have much time to worry about anything else. The anesthesiologist told her to count backwards from 10 and she drifted away to the unknown.

Luna awakens in the recovery room slowly. As she is coming to, a young recovery room tech comes over and checks her vitals and asks how she is feeling. She waits a few seconds and replies that honestly, she cant feel anything at all. He said it was likely from the nerve block they did for pain control when she goes home and it should last approximately two days. Thankful to know that, she nods and closes her eyes. She is so tired, but the recovery techs keep asking questions and trying to keep her awake so they can get her out and back up to her room as soon as possible. After about two hours of answering mundane questions, she finally gets to go back to her room and sleep the anesthesia off. Over the course of the next twenty four hours or so, Luna was in a haze. Every time she opened her eyes it seemed, they were putting pain medication into her IV. She wasn't complaining though, by any means. She wished she could take the whole IV pole and pain meds home with her. Honestly, she was terrified to go home, terrified that when the meds wore off she would feel that searing pain and not be able to handle it. The following morning they came in with breakfast and woke her up to try and eat. They informed her that she was being discharged soon and that PT would be in shortly to get her up into the chair for a little while. Luna could not believe it and started to panic, the nurse said it was common practice and she would be ok.

PT came in a few minutes later and got her up and she sat in the chair for about an hour but she was nauseated the whole time. She called David and let him know that she was coming home today and to make arrangements to pick her up within the next few hours. He sounded almost as panicked as she was. Neither of them knew how home life was going to play out as their bedroom was up a flight of steps about eighteen high and once up, she would not be able to come down on her own. Dr Sanderson came by and went over the surgery details and said that it seems that everything went as planned and gave her the aftercare instructions and some light PT exercises to do from home. David arrives a little while later and has his friend with him to help get her home and up the stairs. After signing the discharge paperwork and watching him gather all of her belongings that were going with them, Luna was helped into a wheelchair and left the hospital for the first time in a little over a week.

After stopping at the pharmacy and picking up her antibiotics, anti inflammatories and pain medication, they finally arrived at the house and that's where the real challenges were faced. Between the two men, they were able to get Luna upstairs and settled into bed. Just that small amount of activity wore her out and before long she was fast asleep. The next few weeks were an opiate induced blur for her. The surgeon sent her home on Percocet 10mg but they were not taking her pain away so she had been given permission to double the dose and *double the dose she did*. She did not care if the house fell apart on top of her as long as she was not in pain. Bills piled up & the house was a mess but Luna did not care about any of that. She took her pills and slept. She much preferred the utopia to reality nowadays. David, Zoe and Blake learned to take care of themselves in addition to taking care of her. She needed help with the simplest tasks as she was not allowed to bear weight on her foot. To get downstairs was a complete joke. Their bedroom, much like her hospital room, had become her new home.

During this time, she and David really started clashing and having more and more arguments. He turned into someone she did not know anymore and started making hateful comments and she could tell that he was getting weary of "taking care of her." He made her feel useless most of the time and their relationship was really struggling. She knew he was at his breaking point when he snapped at her and threw a container of ice cream at her because she did not want to eat it out of the container, she wanted it in a cup, with milk. She felt that after all the years they had been together that he should have known by now how she liked it and he was just being lazy. David started drinking pretty heavily and was throwing parties at the house while Luna could only stay in her room. They had a steady stream of visitors coming and going almost daily. The kids were grossly unsupervised and were getting into trouble at school often. She felt helpless. After a few weeks though, Luna started to become less affected by the pain meds, they still took her pain away but they did not make her sleep all the time. She was able to function for the most part. She was even able to walk around the room with her crutches as long as she was careful not to let that foot touch the floor. She took a few falls and three broken toes before she learned how to navigate correctly on them but getting up and moving was worth it. At least she could get up in the morning and watch the kids walk out and down to the bus stop now, she would smile and wave at them every morning. She also finally figured out that she could toss her crutches down the stairs and go down on her rear end to the rolling chair waiting at the bottom. This would be good because now she can spend more time with the kids and keep a better eye on them. She went down that first morning and was stunned. The kitchen looked as if it had not been cleaned in a month. There were dirty dishes overflowing the sink and onto the countertops. The trash was so full you could not get another thing into it. Food boxes and empathy containers were everywhere. She sat there in her rolling chair just staring at the utter filth in shock. All she wanted was a sandwich.

There was not even any room on the countertops to make one.

Luna grabbed her crutches and stood carefully on the kitchen floor and decided to at least try to do something. She started grabbing trash and stuffing it into the already full can. As she was doing so, her crutch slipped and she went down face first, hitting her head on the wall as she went. Her cast bounced off the floor several times and she thought her knees were going to explode. Crying and in so much pain, she could only lay there trying to figure out how she was going to get up. David was "gone fishing" and the kids were over at friends houses. She called Zoe, she was the closest. Zoe told her not to move and she would come home in less than ten minutes. When she arrived, her and her friend were able to help Luna into a standing position and sit her back in her chair and ask why she was even downstairs to begin with. Luna, still crying, said: "I just wanted a sandwich!" This set Zoe and her friend into a fit of giggles and eventually Luna joined in, half crying, half laughing, as they cleared off a spot on the countertop and fixed her a sandwich.

They then set to work cleaning up a little bit so that Luna would not attempt it again. When the kitchen wasn't "so disgusting" anymore, they asked if she needed anything else and offered to help her back upstairs but she declined and asked if they would fetch a pain pill and then she'd be ok. They left and went back to her friend's house while Luna spent some time downstairs for the first time in a while. She sat outside on the deck for hours soaking in the sunshine that her face had not seen in what felt like a very, very long time. After she had her fill of sunshine, she wheeled herself back to the stairs and went up, backwards, on her rear. Then she had a real bath for the first time in what must have been a month (with her right leg hanging out) and it was the most glorious bath ever. She washed and conditioned her hair twice and she must have stayed in that tub for over two hours! She dried herself the best she could and crawled back in the cozy comfort of her bed.

Feeling almost human again, Luna was finally feeling a little more hopeful.

Until she went to her follow up appointment. Her surgeon cut off her cast and took x-rays and she wasn't healing as well as he had planned so he recasted the foot and added more time to the "non-weight bearing" orders. It was disappointing but there was nothing she could do about it except to follow doctors orders. Luna ended up spending a total of twelve weeks in the cast and on crutches, then another eight weeks in a walking boot that the kids called "Robo-Boot." About three or four more weeks went by and she got to ditch the boot and finally, she was permitted to get back to work. She was allowed to drive now that the boot was gone and life seemed to get back to a new version of normal. She and David were really growing apart though. He spent more and more time away from home with any excuse he could find. Luna did not know what to do and just allowed him his space now that she was a little more independant. She still had a fair amount of pain, however, it was controllable as long as she took her meds as scheduled.

Once she started working again she lost her medical assistance which was unfortunate because she was supposed to have her hardware removed in a month. One day, Luna was in her closet looking for clothes to wear to work the following day and eyeing her favorite wedge sandals, she decided to try them on and see if they would fit. With her foot unable to bend at certain angles now though, she quickly found out that this would not be a possibility now or in the future. She sat there on the closet floor crying as Zoe helped her go through all of her footwear and throw about fifteen pairs of shoes into a donation bag. This was when her depression started hitting pretty hard. Eventually the doctor decided it was time to wean her from the opiate based pain pills. He gradually took her from 20mg to 10mg to 5mg then took her off the percocet entirely and gave her a non-narcotic pain medicine which did not help at all. She begged her doctor to at least put her on a low dose and keep her on it but he refused.

This is the point when Luna started looking elsewhere for relief.
She would buy them from friends, family and even strangers for the next few years. She developed heavy anxiety issues at the thought of being in pain if she stopped taking them altogether but eventually, her resources ran dry and she could no longer keep herself supplied. In desperation, Luna sought out a different doctor who took down her symptoms and did an exam.

He diagnosed her with peripheral neuropathy and arthritis in that leg and foot. Neuropathy, she found out, is just a fancy name for nerve damage. The pain she had been feeling, the heat and shocks/stabs were all from the injury and the surgery. He put her back on some actual pain medication which couldn't have made her happier. He kept her on them for about a year before the FDA and DEA started the "war on opiates" and cracked down on doctors prescribing opioid painkillers. Since her hardware had never been removed there was a fair amount of scar tissue that grew around it and was contributing to her pain. Because of that and the neuropathy, he referred her to a pain management clinic but Luna declined. She had made the decision to finally try to get off of the painkillers. Thinking about her mother, who was an addict Luna's whole life, she could not imagine herself becoming like her. Ever. And if she continued on like this, she most certainly would. It was at this point in her thoughts that her mind slipped back to when she was twelve years old. *Here, she relives it like a slap in the face.*

59

Chapter 5 (Reliving Trauma)

When she was fifteen months old, her father and mother divorced. Since she was the youngest child and hadn't "bonded" with her mother like her sister had, Luna's father took her when he left. She does not remember any of this, just what she was told over the years. Her father and step-mother (Barbara) raised her from a baby. She was the only child in the household but not the "only" child. She had an older sister that she saw periodically and also had three step-sisters that she saw on a regular basis. She sometimes felt like they treated her with contempt because their mother left them for her father, and she was raising Luna instead of her own children so of course she understood if there were hard feelings. She never understood this until she was an adult and these feelings were admitted to her by one of them. She remembers that they moved a lot when she was young. Memories of one state get blurred between memories of another. She recalls going to primary school in Georgia. They moved between Atlanta, Acworth, Lavonia and Villa Rica when Luna was very small. She liked Acworth and Villa Rica the most.

She loved going to the racetrack with her dad on the weekends. Coming home covered in red Georgia clay dust from the track. She has very fond memories of those times. Then, in Villa Rica she recalls the house in vivid detail. The garden outside, the pecan trees and the pond that always froze over in the winter-time. It was a wonderland for a child. Luna and Jade spent a lot of time outdoors playing make-believe. There was a huge cornfield that separated their house and the neighbors. She doesn't remember seeing the house, only that massive cornfield she and Jade would play in for hours on end. They drank from water hoses and dug in the dirt until it was dark. Barbara would hose them off before coming into the house when they had been playing in the mud. These were wonderful memories as well. The garden out back was dad's PTSD therapy garden. He spent hours there after work, tending the vegetables. There were watermelons, tomatoes, cucumbers, squash, cabbage and rows of green beans. Barbara spent a fair amount of time in the kitchen canning and storing vegetables for the winter. In the fall, they would all be sent outside with pillowcases to gather the fallen pecans, these were also canned and stored.

The pond on their property would freeze up and if they were careful, they could ice skate in the winter.

She does recall falling in a few times but it was not deep so there was never any real danger. Despite all of this sounding like a fairy-tale, this was when her memories of the fighting really kicked in between dad and Barbara. They could be heard in the middle of the night screaming at each other through the walls of Luna's room sometimes. During the day time fights, she would frequently hide in a laundry hamper with the clothes pulled on top of herself and the lid closed. It scared her so bad. He had the worst temper with her it seemed. She recalls the fights, the yelling, and the frequent whippings that she would receive when she was a "klutz" or when she would get a nosebleed and bleed all over her step-mothers linens. Looking back, she thinks that it was those fights that would make Barbara be mean to her sometimes. Like the time that she tripped over the fan cord and Barbara chased her outside and beat her rear pretty good and pulled some of her hair out. She remembers standing there on the back porch, crying, running her hands through her hair and casting the clumps off the deck as she silently berated herself for her clumsiness. She only recalls a few of these moments though. Her daddy was her whole life. He was her entire world.

She could not understand why he would get so angry and scream at Barbara for seemingly no reason. Every now and then he would yell at Luna too but she can only recollect him whipping her once when she was young and she knew she deserved it. She had lied about getting a demerit in class and tried to hide the call from her teacher. He sat and cried afterwards as he hugged her. Luna knew without a doubt that he loved her very much. When she turned eighteen and her step-mom gave her his belongings she found out a lot about him that she never knew. He was a Vietnam Vet. He had PTSD, schizophrenic episodes, Acute Neurosis and Delusions of Grandeur. That explained a lot of his behavior towards her step-mom to her. What she does remember of her earlier times with Barbara is that she did love Luna. Regardless of her "moments" she loved and cared for her like she was her own.
At some point, they left that house and moved to a condo in Florida. This was where they were all the happiest. They had a large fenced-in backyard and a little springer spaniel puppy to

run around. Dad was an electrician and Barbara worked in the printing industry. She would bring Luna home stickers, sticker books and coloring books galore. She had so many toys and books that she was always occupied.

She went after school to gymnastics and after that she was bussed over to the boys and girls club where she was on the swim team. They had many activities like art classes, jazzercise and tutors that helped with homework. She had a full schedule before dad picked her up to go home. At the house, there was an orange tree in the front that they often traded with the neighbor for his grapefruit on the tree in his yard. Their neighbor to the left was an old man who had a pet squirrel and sometimes he would even let Luna feed it peanuts. Brian and his parents lived on the right and he was her best friend in the world. They were always riding their bikes together and playing outside, exploring the neighborhood and getting into all sorts of mischief. There was also a pool in the neighborhood to swim. Barbara loved the beach and they spent a lot of time there also. Splashing in the waves and building sandcastles with anyone who wanted to join in. The sun was always shining and life seemed to be going so good.

Until her daddy died. It happened so suddenly, she was there in the house when he suffered a massive aneurysm in his brain. Luna had just walked into the kitchen to grab a drink when her dad started screaming. Holding his head and crying, running aimlessly through the living room. She will never forget that moment. The look of pure terror on her step-mom's face, her screaming over him and begging him to tell her what was wrong, what was happening, while frantically grabbing her purse and keys before ushering him to the car. She yelled out the window as she drove away that she would call someone to come and to lock the door and wait. He was brain-dead before they reached the hospital. Luna was left standing in shock in the middle of the kitchen, wondering what was happening to her dad. Her aunt arrived and stayed with her that night. The following morning Barbara called and asked them to come to the hospital. They arrived as the doctor was in there talking to her and let her know that he was not going to recover from this and would be on life support until she made a decision. Her aunt fainted and had to be revived with smelling salts. This was another core memory.

To this day, Luna cannot smell ammonia without seeing him laying there with tubes and wires coming from every part of his once strong body. It hit her at that moment that she would never feel his hugs or have him grab her knees and tickle her until she thought she would pee her pants. She would never see him smile again or hear his voice. She would never feel the wind ripping through her skin as she held him tight from the back of his motorcycle. Her daddy was dead. He spent three days in a vegetative-coma before Barbara was given a choice to "pull the plug". It was the single most horrifying and traumatic event of little Luna's entire childhood. This is why Luna often says that her life both ended and began at that moment. The next few days were hazy. She can barely remember the ride back to Georgia. They flew his body back on a plane and they drove. They stayed a night with some family in Tampa and Luna still dont even know who it was. She couldn't function. She remembers hearing the word "catatonic" used to describe her state of being several times by different people but could not tell you who it was or why. It felt like she was sleepwalking, just going in the direction in which she was guided by unseen hands. She can't even recall the funeral in detail.

She remembers a few faces and signing a register book that was laying open by the front door as everyone else seemed to be doing so. But she can't remember ever seeing her father in the casket.

After her father died, Barbara fought tooth and nail for Luna, and lost. All of a sudden, at the wake after his funeral, Luna was forced (by law) to move in with her birth mother, Lisa. At twelve years old she had lost her father, and now was losing the only mother she had ever known. She showed up at Luna's grandmother's house with the police and her birth certificate and they made her go home with Lisa. It was like a horrible nightmare. Unbeknownst to anyone, Lisa was an addict. Luna gets there and her entire way of life is altered. Her older sister, Rachel and little (half-brother) Charlie were not very welcoming. She was virtually a stranger to them and even though they knew they were family, they didn't really know each other as family should. Luna was an "upset" in their life. She was a competition for affection. And she was literally a freshly traumatized mess. She never thought of herself as overly innocent or naïve until she moved into that place, even though she obviously was. Her new step-dad (Will) was very nice. He worked for the FAA and tried his hardest to accept this "new" member of the family. He was polite, giving, and never mean to her. Little by little though, She came to realize that her mother and sister were not normal. They were very secretive.

They whispered a lot, and they hid things from everyone. Finally, she realized why. They were meth addicts (crank, back in the day). Luna's sister was fourteen and already an addict. Rachel teased her relentlessly. All of the pent up hatred she had throughout her childhood because her "daddy loved Luna so much more" came down on Luna's head every single day at first it seemed. She felt guilty and ashamed. It wasn't HER fault that daddy took her and not her sister but you couldn't make Rachel understand that. She called her "daddy's princess" & "spoiled princess." They made fun of Luna at the dinner table because she couldn't cut her own meat. When she cried and said that Barbara always cut it for her, they laughed. They took her knife and made her eat with her hands because she was making a mess trying to cut it herself. Eventually, she learned that if she kissed up and did what they said that they all got along much better. One day Lisa walked in the living room while Will was in the shower and flipped his checkbook open and snatched a check out. Luna watched her from her spot on the sofa, not knowing what was going on. Lisa looked at her and said "go ahead and tell him, I know you are" Well, she did. She didn't really have a reason to or even know what she was doing was wrong until Lisa said that and she hated her for that contemptuous voice. Just the way she said it struck a nerve. Lisa and Will fought about it and he looked further into his finances and noticed that Lisa had been doing this for a very long time and they ended up divorcing very soon after that. Luna WAS TO BLAME for that. Oh well, what more can she do? They were now alone. Mother, sister, brother and herself. Luna eventually looked up to her sister, she was older and wiser. She's the one who gave Luna her first line of meth. After that...well...she was addicted. Rachel's the one who pushed her into losing her virginity at thirteen years old. She teased her and called her names until she finally did it. After it was over, Luna found out that Rachel and her boyfriend were watching the whole time through the window from the roof, to see if she really went through with it. They were allowed to do pretty much whatever they wanted because the five hundred and eighty dollar social security check that their mom got for Luna and the five hundred and twenty dollar check that she got for Rachel, since dad died, kept Lisa supplied really well with her meth each month. Some say that it's the only reason why she fought to get custody of Luna when he died. For the money. She now believes them.

This was a different world for her. She had way too much freedom. And with freedom at that age, you can imagine a scene they made.

Rachel and Luna soon became inseparable. They ran amuck in the small town that they lived in. Drinking, doing drugs and having sex with anyone and everyone they wanted. They had no reservations about sneaking out at night and running the streets. They even hitchhiked sometimes with truck drivers to friends' houses. One day, one of Rachel's friends, Jennifer, told her that she and her parents were going to Florida for a week. Rachel went to Luna's room that night and said "We are going to go break in her house" and they did. They dressed themselves up in all black, gloves and all, and walked down the dirt road to her house and robbed them blind. It was the most horrible feeling in the world, even for someone of such a young age, the conscience was there. When they returned, they were in Rachel's bedroom going through their "loot" when Lisa walked in on the two of them. Immediately, Luna jumped up and started trying to hide the evidence. Rachel just sat there. Lisa asked what was going on and Rachel told her. Unfazed, their mother says "Did you get the VCR?" Luna was shocked! She sent them back to the scene of the crime for the VCR.

She and Rachel are walking up the dirt road, at two AM, carrying a stolen VCR, it was surreal. It was at that very moment that Luna lost any and all respect that she may have developed for her. She remembers her mom going through the stuff and taking her share. The following morning, Lisa took her and their loot and went to this guy's house, she called him her "front-man". Luna even remembers his name, Jimbo. While she sat in the car waiting, Luna watched Lisa walk up to this man's car, get in and then she saw her head disappear. Even at the young age of thirteen, she knew what her mother was doing and she was angry. She was utterly disgusted. Lisa returned with an 8 ball for herself and two grams of meth each for Luna and Rachel. Luna was so bad on it at that point that she did it during school, in the bathroom stall. She kept her supplies (mirror, razor and drugs) in a tiny velvet bag that came with a Barbie that her dad had gotten her before he passed. She was only in sixth grade and didn't care about anything. Not herself, no one. She was alone and confused. She weighed a mere 64lbs from the drugs. She felt lost. She overdosed on muscle relaxers at school one day. She took these from her grandmother and used them to help "ease her down from the meth". She was suspended for ten days.

School at that point was her only escape. She had a life there, friends. Now, even they are gone. At that moment, she decided that she'd had enough. They were in bad shape at home, had no running water, no gas and no heat. They had a propane heater and a bucket to shit and piss in. The house stank. They all stunk like propane. They were living like total vagabonds and she wasn't used to that. She was a "princess" and her life wasn't supposed to be like this. She had never been without anything in her life that she could recall. She called her step-mom and begged Barbara to come get her. She said she couldn't, that Lisa had full custody of Luna now. She cried and begged to the point that she finally said she would. Barbara told Luna to tell Lisa that she was coming to stay with her for two weeks. So she did, and after a lot of yelling and screaming on both ends, she finally said it was ok. Barbara came and picked her up that day and the moment she sat in her car, she'll never forget, she said **"you stink, omg, what is that smell & what is going on?"** So she talked and she talked and she talked. She spilled everything on that three hour car ride that had happened since she went to live there with Lisa. They were both crying by the time they pulled up at her house.

She made Luna shower and called her daughter, Jade, over to stay with her while she went to see an attorney to file for emergency custody. For the next week, Jade helped Luna through the withdrawals, the nightmares, the cold sweats and all the mood swings that came along with coming off of methamphetamines. She was a mess. She doesn't really remember most of that time but Barbara and Jade told her all about it when it was over. She doesn't know what she would have done without Jade. After the two weeks went by and Luna didn't call or come home, Lisa called and asked what was going on. Luna was cold as ice. She told her that she was now fourteen and finally had the "say-so" over who she wanted to live with and she chose to stay here. Lisa threw a tantrum, called the police and reported her as a runaway. The police swarmed Barbara's home at eight AM that following morning and hauled Luna into the local station as Barbara was at work and there was no paperwork available to show them. She was scared to death. Barbara left work and armed with all the information Luna had given her, names of dealers and such, had already applied for and was granted temporary emergency custody of Luna. Lisa went home empty-handed.

Not only empty-handed but barely escaped being thrown in jail for making such a scene when she was turned away by the officers and attorney. Luna will never forget those words "ma'am, you need to just go home, if you keep on like this we will arrest you for disorderly conduct". Those words were the best she had heard all day.

The day before their court-date, Lisa called and told her that she gave up. Luna could stay, she wouldn't fight any more. She knew that she would be humiliated and lose her in court anyways. Come to find out, Rachel, later that night, called some suicide hotline and told a counselor a bunch of stuff that alerted authorities and DFACS and Lisa went to jail for possession. Rachel ended up in some rehab and Luna's step-dad took Charlie. Boy, she hated Luna at the moment and she really didn't care. She wanted to put that part of her life in the past and try to move on.

Chapter 6 (Moving On)

For the next year or so Luna managed to live a relatively normal teenage life. She tried to date. But all the boys seemed to want was sex. She gave in and had sex with her boyfriend and became really shaky and threw up afterwards. She tried again a few months later and the same thing happened so she gave up on it. She thought she was a freak and *so did he*. He broke up with her, of course and then some time afterwards she started seeing this grown man of thirty two named Pete. She sure thought she was special to be dating an older man. As an adult, looking back, he was nothing but a pedophile. Eventually they split, they couldn't keep it a secret forever. Not long after, Barbara, Luna and Mark (Barbara's fiancee) sold their home and moved to another city where Luna met Chase. She was now close to sixteen years old. He was a bad boy. Exciting. She quickly fell in love. Barbara really hated him though, she said he was shady and after a few months she forbade her to see him. She snuck around and saw him every chance she got though and one day they decided to run away together. Three days went by and the police finally found them. They made Luna go home and she and Barbara got in a huge fight.

Luna ended up on her ass on the bedroom floor. She told her that it was her own choice, that she could live in her house and stop seeing him or she could leave and do whatever she wanted. Well, she thought she knew it all and said she was not going to stop seeing him.

Barbara, in a fit of rage, gave Luna until midnight to gather her stuff and get out. She called Chase but couldn't stay with him, of course. So she called her aunt Diane and she took her in. She quit school and got a job with Diane at a laundromat and lived there pretty peacefully for about a year. Then one night, her son (Luna's cousin) came banging on her window at three AM begging her to let him in, the front door was locked and he was drunk. So she did.. already drunk, he sat there on the floor of her bedroom with a bottle of wild turkey and they talked, laughed, cried and drank till she was completely shit-faced. He then raped her. Brutally. She was so drunk that she couldn't even scream, it came out as gurgles. She couldn't move, she was on her stomach and puked in her bed as he was doing it. She passed out before it was over. When she awoke, in a pool of her own vomit, he was gone. Luna was quiet for weeks, withdrawn, trying to piece together in her head what the hell she had done

to deserve that. She was so ashamed, gross and dirty. He was her cousin for god's sake. Why had he done this to her? That was the first time out of three, he did it every chance he could get. Once in the kitchen with his hand over her mouth, and twice after they moved to a smaller home, he crept into her bedroom that she shared with her grandmother and woke her up with a hand over her mouth, his voice through gritted teeth daring her to scream & wake their granny up. She kept her mouth shut for months, not knowing who to talk to, who she could trust or who would "save her." She was a wreck and she felt so alone in her own head. She was ruined. *Emotionally, Luna completely shut down.*
Her aunt asked what was bothering her but she couldn't tell her. She didn't want to, she was so ashamed and uncomfortable telling Diane what her own son had done to her. So she broke down and called Barbara and begged her to come get her AGAIN. She did, of course. She was always there for Luna. Diane eventually found out and their relationship was never the same after that. Another person lost to her. She tried to go on with her life, Barbara re-enrolled her in high school but she really wasn't interested. She felt like she was too far behind.

All the trivial things that were "high-school" were childish to her now. She was an adult and had seen and done too much to be placed back in "day-care" so she piddled along and played the school game for as long as she could before running into Chase again. He was her first love. He was all she ever wanted. She took a summer course and graduated high school early and immediately got pregnant. Barbara called the abortion clinic from the health department as soon as the test came back positive and set her up for an abortion, she was still a minor in HER household. It was a whirlwind. Luna cried and protested but "mom's word was law." She wasn't given a choice, even though it was her body and her life. The next morning, she was lying on a table, unconscious, having an abortion. That night, as she was laying there cramping and bleeding, crying and mourning the loss of the child she no longer had inside, she picked up the bottle of Percocet lying beside her and took twelve of them. Hoping to just die. She didn't, she couldn't even do that right. She woke up the next morning and as soon as her feet hit the floor, she did too, face first. She vomited until she thought she WOULD die. She told Jade what she had done and Jade immediately ran and told Barbara.

She walked in the bathroom and stood there looking at Luna and said "I don't have time for your games, I have to work" And she left. Luna was floored. Totally ashamed and embarrassed. Jade called her boyfriend who came and sat with her as Kara and Mary took her to the hospital where they pumped what was left from her stomach and admitted her on a "1013" suicide watch. After her evaluation from the hospital psychologist and a few days of observation they released her into Barbara's care and they went home. Again, Life Goes On. She tried to get Luna some psychological help and put her into counseling after her insurance wouldn't pay for in-patient care. However, she was unresponsive to treatment. She felt no one understood, she was closed up. Locked tight. She had no control over anything and she felt invisible, like her voice did not matter, she just wanted to die. One day Barbara came home from work and told her that she was going nowhere; she was 17, and needed to figure life out. If she didn't do something now, she was never going to be anything. She talked to her and got her a job at the printing company that she managed. She had given up on trying to stop her from seeing Chase and things were going good.

Then one day, out of the blue.. Barbara came home and sat Luna and Jade down and talked to them. She informed them that she had done all she could. She was done. She was tired. She said that it was time to think of herself for once and that she was moving to her lake house that she went to on the weekends. For good. She said that it was time for Jade and Luna to grow up and figure things out on their own. She gave them a month to do so. Jade (who was 16) married Tony. Chase and Luna moved in with her other step-sister Mary. Luna was still working at the printing company and not long after she turned 18, found out she was pregnant again, with Zoe. She pretty much had her shit as together as well as she could at that age so she and Chase got married. By then, they had been together off and on since she was fifteen and it was expected anyways. Mary had said that she would not let them continue to live under her roof unless they were married either. It was a horrible marriage. Turns out, he wasn't her "Prince Charming" after all. All they ever did was fight over sex mainly, she didn't want it, he did. He was rough. He was uncaring. He became mentally and physically abusive because he was bi-polar and had started using drugs. He cheated and lied and after giving him a thousand "chances" Luna gave up. She was mentally checked out of the marriage already.

The day that she caught him shooting up meth was the last day we were together. She took Zoe and walked out the door. Zoe was barely four years old when they divorced. He was an addict and she had sworn that she would never live her life with a meth addict again and she meant that. She moved in with her other step-sister Kara at that time and she & Zoe thrived. All they had was each other and they were as close as two peas in a pod. Months went by and they were happy, free and loving life. Luna dated a few guys but no one lasted more than a few months. At the time, Jade and Tony were also going through an ugly divorce and on the night of Tony's birthday he called Luna and asked if she wanted to go to a club with him and party. She agreed. They proceeded to get drunk as hell, high on coke and slept together. Not her most shining moment and definitely a horrible decision. He filled her drugged head with all these things that sounded good to her. He said that he loved her and always had, and that Jade was a mistake and he wished it had been them together instead. This started Luna's newfound love affair with cocaine, and him.

After about a month of sneaking around and finding excuses to be together he asked Luna to take him out of state for a "ball tournament" so she jumped at the chance and they left. In the car, he told her that there was no tournament and he just wanted to get her and Zoe away for the weekend. They knew that the family would have issues with them being together. She knew it was wrong as hell. They should not be anything more than what they started out as, he was her brother-in-law. But he was very convincing. He wanted to marry her and was not taking no for an answer. Despite knowing better, Luna let him take the lead and gave in.

While they were up there, Jade traced his call that he made to their daughter somehow and called the hotel and found the room was registered to Luna. Game Over. Jade and their cousin went into Luna's and Zoe's room at Kara's house and burned almost all of her clothes, cut the straps on all of her shoes and wrote "whore" on her bed, walls, everything, in bright red nail polish. They ruined everything she had. They came to the hotel and called them out. There was almost a fight. It was horrible, even though Jade and Luna stopped being step-sisters the day Luna's father died, she still considered her a SISTER and Luna had wronged Jade in the worst way possible. Worst of all, Luna agreed.

She and Tony couldn't come home. She was so ashamed. Basically exiled from their family, they got a little place out of state for about a month and when he couldn't find work they packed up and moved to his parents in Mississippi. She wasn't quite a "welcome" guest there either. His mother and sister were very short with her and voiced their disapproval of their relationship. It was a very tense living arrangement but he was their son and so they were taken in. Then his sister got into a really bad car accident and Luna was the only one available to take care of her. With the training and experience she had from working at the nursing home as a CNA while she and Chase were married, she was able to bathe his sister and care for her and "earn" her utmost respect. Things were not as tense after that. Luna got pregnant again shortly thereafter. Zoe was only four and a half. Immediately, **for some reason**, she said that she wanted an abortion. That was the answer. The only answer to this problem. He didn't argue, he took her and she had one, in a run-down chop-shop in Jackson Mississippi. They didn't even give her anything for sedation or anesthesia. She screamed so loud from the pain that the nurse yelled at her and told her to "shut up, she was scaring the other patients." She was in an open room and when she looked in front of her, she could see other women having abortions also. It was horrible but LIFE GOES ON. And it did. They stayed there for four months before moving on. They came back home to Georgia and moved in with his grandparents for a short time and then got their own place two houses down from them. Luna wasn't allowed to work. He was "the man" and would take care of them. That was a joke. They lived day-to-day, not even week to week. He developed a huge drug problem, started out with marijuana then progressed to meth and crack. She tolerated it because she felt she deserved this, this was her karma. He and Zoe didn't always get along well, he wasn't really nice to her all the time and he was very strict. He would lock Zoe out of the house so he could do his drugs. Luna would go out there and keep her company. She hated the way he was to her and would baby her in his absence to make up for his treatment. Zoe's father hadn't had much to do with her since Tony and she were together and Luna's heart broke for her baby girl. She wanted to leave him so bad but she had nowhere to go.

They had burned so many bridges that even her own family wouldn't take her in (she thought.)

Chapter 7 (Soulless)

Soon, she was pregnant again. Another abortion. This time she went to where Barbara had taken her. Peaceful and sedated. Four months later... pregnant again. Another abortion. By this time, Luna had started using meth also, on the weekends, as her way of dealing with everything she had been through and was still going through. Plus, it was about the only way she could tolerate him or even being alive. She did not feel worthy of life. Her soul was *destroyed*. She begged and pleaded for him to take her to the health department and let her get on birth control. This was crazy, she couldn't keep having abortions. It was literally making her insane. It hurt to have sex. Sex was truly not enjoyable, it was a chore that she allowed him every other night because if she didn't, he was a complete asshole. He said ok and finally she got on birth control. But he had to go with her and make sure the doctor was a woman because no other man was going to be looking at his "goods." Six months later, somehow, she was pregnant again. Zoe was five now, almost six. Rumors were flying that Luna had cheated on Tony with Chase. No doubt, they were started by Jade.

Everyone was saying that it wasn't his baby and she knew it was. She had never cheated. He didn't let her out of his sight long enough for her to even talk to another man. He demanded that she have this baby and truth be known, she wanted this one. She was so tired of the crap and thought that maybe a baby would change him.

Blake was born and there was no denying that he was Tony's. When Blake was four months old, Luna got pregnant again. Another abortion. By the time she was twenty-five she had killed five babies. She had had enough and it ate a hole in her soul. Mentally, she was hanging on by a thread. Tony eventually went to prison for fraud/forgery from a scheme that he and his friends had cooked up and Luna moved to a place in a small town, just her and the kids. She went in to the doctor with hopes of getting her tubes tied but instead they found cancer cells in her cervix and she had to have a hysterectomy. Good enough reason for her. She was on her own. Two kids with two different fathers. She was broken, used and abused. No family to rely on. He had burned bridges with every move he made. She stayed with him for a year while he was incarcerated. She worked, paid the outlandish jail-phone bills and tried to make it. Then, she woke up. She finally left him.

A few months later she met Adam. He was so nice and sweet and funny. So good to her kids and they had the best time together. It was time for her to move on. She let him move in with her and within six months they were engaged. Life was so very good, finally. Then, Adam got appendicitis. He had emergency surgery and had to stay home for about two or three weeks and lost his job. So, Luna suggested that he just stay home and watch the kids. Save her from paying the $200 a week that she was paying in daycare costs.
Blake was three by this time and Adam agreed to do that. One day Luna came home from work and pulled in the driveway and immediately heard the screaming. She cut the engine and quietly walked up to the front door which was open and saw him standing over the sofa screaming at Zoe and Blake. Zoe had the covers pulled over their heads and both she and Blake were crying. Luna asked what the hell was going on and he saw her and said "these damn kids, they don't listen to a word I say!" She came in and calmed the kids, then went to the room to talk to him. She told him that if She EVER caught him screaming at her kids like that again that he would be out on his ass. About a month later, she woke up early one morning and

gathered the kids while he was sleeping and they went to Shoney's as a treat. While they were there, Blake (being 3) was climbing all over the booth and she noticed a bruise on his back. Zoe was beside him so she asked her to lift his shirt and let her see his back. Luna was mortified. It was a bruise that covered his whole little back! She grabbed the kids, paid the bill and went to her sisters where she undressed Blake and saw other bruises on his legs and testicles. She questioned him as best as she could question a three year old child and he said that Adam hit him. GAME OVER. Luna left her sister's house and went straight to the police station. Within a few hours he was arrested and taken from their home. He was charged with child abuse and the arresting officer was Luna's best friend's mom so she made sure that all of the inmates knew why he was there. She didn't see nor hear from him till the court date a year and a half later. She was questioned because the bruises were a few days old but she explained to them that Blake and Zoe were usually bathed and in their pajamas by the time she got home from work so all she had to do was put them to bed. Blake went through therapy and has since forgotten or blocked the incident. His father was still in prison at the time and when he finally got out, he moved to Texas. Alone again. The kids and Luna lived alone for almost a year before Chase re-entered her life. He gave her this big story about how he had amended his ways and wanted his family back. She took him back. About five months later she started suspecting that he was still using drugs. She called his probation officer and tipped her off and he was arrested for a dirty test the next time he saw her. Luna didn't care, she was so tired of it all, all of the stupid lies and deceit. She packed his stuff and took it to his friend's house. When Blake was six or seven she found Jon. He was her sister Rachel's neighbor. They were perfect together in every way. He was so funny! He absolutely adored the kids. They moved in together after a few months and were engaged about a year later. He worked nights and Luna was in nursing school in the day time though and that eventually put a strain on the relationship. They really only had the weekends together and then his mom was soon diagnosed with cancer. Between that and the pressures of buying a home, he became impotent. He had a lot on his plate. He and Luna were not intimate for eight whole months. She thought it was her, maybe she was not attractive anymore. He did not tell her what was going on due to his own embarrassment.

They drifted apart because she thought all kinds of bad stuff and never thought for one second that it was him, not her. She met someone online and ended up cheating on Jon. He accepted it somehow. He knew that he had pushed Luna away and wanted to work it out. He begged her to stay and work through things, he really was a good man. To this day, he and Luna are still in touch, he still claims the kids as his step-children and he is still quite a good man. Blake and Jon are very close and he thinks of him as a father figure since his own father is not in his life. He didn't deserve what she did to him and she should have stayed. But she didn't. She was with David now and was going to live happily ever after…lol. For the first three years things were great, and then he cheated on Luna with his boss. This happened right before the wreck and they had been trying to get past it but things were never really the same after that. He started doing a lot of different pills during Luna's recovery and she was becoming sure he was developing a problem. She had contacted a personal injury attorney to see if anything could be done for the pain she would have the rest of her life and received a large settlement from the wreck. Once the check finally arrived, David demanded "his share."

Confused, Luna asked what exactly he was referring to as he had not been in the wreck or suffered any injuries. He said that he felt he should be compensated for his time taking care of her after the wreck. In absolute awe at his audacity, Luna made the decision to end the farce of a relationship they had, bought him a new car and sent him packing. She had done plenty of personal growth and knew that she deserved better than that. This officially brings Luna's story to a close.

EPILOGUE

Every day was a constant struggle and she did not always stay on the right path but eventually she was able to get used to the pain and find ways to ease it. She found that a TENS unit helped on the really bad days. Luna has dated several other guys after David but none could handle the fact that she doesn't like to leave her home much unless it's to go to work and back. Looking back, this was the cause of many failed relationships. After many years of recovery, Luna has found that between the gradual weight gain, anxiety and pain, she has turned herself into a virtual recluse. The weight gain was caused by her now inactive lifestyle. This was not a choice, she used to really enjoy outings and activities. But she no longer enjoys going out with friends and prefers small and more private gatherings to large crowds. Her anxiety makes sure she stays out of any trouble.. (funny stuff right there!) While her friends and family all enjoy hiking, camping, going to the river in the summertime, kayaking, trips to fairs and theme parks, Luna just can't. Even a trip to the grocery store for weekly groceries hurts. Being on her foot for more than an hour at a time causes significant pain and swelling. The chiropractor did x-rays and said he did not understand how she even functioned on a day to day basis. This is what chronic pain does to a person. It shapes their whole being into something else. She has honestly just accepted the pain, fear and anxiety and lives with it now. It is a part of her life and who she is. Luna calls it her "darkness" and she currently lives her life in relative isolation, if anything, it's peaceful there.

The End

www.ingramcontent.com/pod-product-compliance
Lightning Source LLC
Chambersburg PA
CBHWC70252220526
45465CB00004B/1590